No. 2---University Series.

THE

CORRELATION

OF

Vital and Physical Forces.

BY PROF. GEO. F. BARKER, M.D.,
Yale College.

NEW HAVEN, CONN.:
CHARLES C. CHATFIELD.
1870.

New Haven, Conn.:
The College Courant Print.

The Correlation

of

Vital and Physical Forces.

In the Syracusan Poecile, says Alexander von Humboldt in his beautiful little allegory of the Rhodian Genius, hung a painting, which, for full a century, had continued to attract the attention of every visitor. In the foreground of this picture a numerous company of youths and maidens of earthly and sensuous appearance gazed fixedly upon a haloed Genius who hovered in their midst. A butterfly rested upon his shoulder, and he held in his hand a flaming torch. His every lineament bespoke a celestial origin. The attempts to solve the enigma of this painting—whose origin even was unknown—though numerous, were all in vain, when one day a ship arriving from Rhodes, laden with works of art, brought another picture, at once recognized as its companion. As before, the Genius stood in the center, but the butterfly had disappeared, and the torch was reversed and extinguished. The youths and maidens were no longer sad and submissive, their mutual embraces announcing their entire emancipation from restraint. Still unable to solve the riddle, Dionysius sent the pictures to the Pythagorean sage, Epicharmus. After gazing upon them long and earnestly, he said : Sixty years long have I pondered on the internal springs of nature, and on the differences inherent in matter; but it is only this day that the Rhodian Genius has taught me to see clearly that which before I had only conjectured. In inanimate nature, everything seeks its like. Everything, as soon as formed, hastens to enter into new combinations, and nought save the disjoining art of man can present in a separate state ingredients which ye would vainly seek in the interior of the earth or in the moving oceans of air and water. Different, however, is the blending of the same substances in animal and vegetable bodies. Here vital force imperatively asserts its rights, and heedless of the affinity and antagonism of the atoms, unites substances which in inanimate nature ever flee from each other, and separates that which is incessantly striving to unite. Recognize, therefore, in the Rhodian Genius, in the expression of his youthful vigor, in the butterfly on his shoulder, in the commanding glance of his eye, the symbol of vital force as it animates every germ of organic creation. The earthly elements at his feet are striving to gratify their own desires and to mingle with one another. Imperiously the Genius threatens them with upraised and high-flaming torch, and compels them regardless of their ancient rights, to obey his laws. Look now on the new work of art; turn from life to death. The butterfly has soared upward, the extinguished torch is reversed, and the head of the youth is drooping; the spirit has fled to other spheres, and the vital force is extinct. Now the youths and maidens join their hands in joyous accord. Earthly matter again resumes its rights. Released from all bonds, they impetuously follow their natural instincts, and the day of his death is to them a day of nuptials.[1]

The view here put by Humboldt into the mouth of Epicharmus may be taken as a fair representation of the current opinion of all ages concerning vital force. To-day, as truly as seventy-five years ago when Humboldt wrote, the mysterious and awful phenomena of life are commonly attributed to some controlling agent residing in the organism—to some independent presiding deity, holding it in absolute subjection. Such a notion it was which prompted Heraclitus to talk of a universal fire, Van Helmont to propose his Archæus, Hofmann his vital fluid, Hunter his *materia vitæ diffusa*, and Humboldt his vital force.[2] All these names assume the existence of a material or immaterial something, more or less separable from the material body, and more or less identical with the mind or soul, which is the cause of the phenomena of living beings. But as science moved irresistibly onward, and it became evident that the forces of inorganic nature were neither deities nor imponderable fluids, separable from matter, but were simple affections of it, analogy demanded a like concession in behalf of vital force.[3] From the notion that the effects of heat were due to an imponderable fluid called caloric, discovery passed to the conviction that heat was but a motion of material particles, and hence inseparable from matter. To a like assumption concerning vitality it was now but a step. The more advanced thinkers in science of to-day, therefore, look upon the life of the living form as inseparable from its substance, and believe that the former is purely phenomenal, and only a manifestation of the latter. Denying the existence of a special vital force as such, they retain the term only to express the sum of the phenomena of living beings.

In calling your attention this evening to the Correlation of the Physical and the Vital Forces, I have a twofold object in view. On the one hand, I would seek to interest you in a comparatively recent discovery of Science, and one which is destined to play a most important part in promoting man's welfare; and on the other I would inquire what part our own country has had in these discoveries.

In the first place, then, let us consider what the evidences are that vital and physical forces are correlated. Let us inquire how far inorganic and organic forces may be considered mutually convertible, and hence, in so far, mutually identical. This may best be done by considering, first, what is to be understood by correlation: and second, how far are the physical forces themselves correlated to each other.

At the outset of our discussion, we are met by an unfortunate ambiguity of language. The word Force, as commonly used, has three distinct meanings; in the first place, it is used to express the cause of motion, as when we speak of the force of gunpowder; it is also used to indicate motion itself, as when we refer to the force of a moving cannon-ball; and lastly it is employed to express the effect of motion, as when we speak of the blow which the moving body gives.[4] Because of this confusion, it has been found convenient to adopt Rankine's suggestion,[5] and to substitute the word 'energy' therefor. And precisely as all force upon the earth's surface—

using the term force in its widest sense—may be divided into attraction and motion, so all energy is divided into potential and actual energy, synonymous with those terms. It is the chemical attraction of the atoms, or their potential energy, which makes gunpowder so powerful; it is the attraction or potential energy of gravitation which gives the power to a raised weight. If now, the impediments be removed, the power just now latent becomes active, attraction is converted into motion, potential into actual energy, and the desired effect is accomplished. The energy of gunpowder or of a raised weight is potential, is capable of acting; that of exploding gunpowder or of a falling weight is actual energy or motion. By applying a match to the gunpowder, by cutting the string which sustains the weight, we convert potential into actual energy. By potential energy, therefore, is meant attraction; and by actual energy, motion. It is in the latter sense that we shall use the word force in this lecture; and we shall speak of the forces of heat, light, electricity and mechanical motion, and of the attractions of gravitation, cohesion, chemism.

From what has now been said, it is obvious that when we speak of the forces of heat, light, electricity or motion, we mean simply the different modes of motion called by these names. And when we say that they are correlated to each other, we mean simply that the mode of motion called heat, light, electricity, is convertible into any of the others, at pleasure. Correlation therefore implies convertibility, and mutual dependence and relationship.

Having now defined the use of the term force, and shown that forces are correlated which are convertible and mutually dependent, we go on to study the evidences of such correlation among the motions of inorganic nature usually called physical forces ; and to ask what proof science can furnish us that mechanical motion, heat, light, and electricity are thus mutually convertible. As we have already hinted, the time was when these forces were believed to be various kinds of imponderable matter, and chemists and physicists talked of the union of iron with caloric as they talked of its union with sulphur, regarding the caloric as much a distinct and inconvertible entity as the iron and sulphur themselves. Gradually, however, the idea of the indestructibility of matter extended itself to force. And as it was believed that no material particle could ever be lost, so, it was argued, no portion of the force existing in nature can disappear. Hence arose the idea of the indestructibility of force. But, of course, it was quite impossible to stop here. If force cannot be lost, the question at once arises, what becomes of it when it passes beyond our recognition ? This question led to experiment, and out of experiment came the great fact of force-correlation ; a fact which distinguished authority has pronounced the most important discovery of the present century.[6] These experiments distinctly proved that when any one of these forces disappeared, another took its place ; that when motion was arrested, for example, heat, light or electricity was developed. In short, that these forces were so intimately related or correlated —to use the word then proposed by Mr. Grove[7]—that when one of them vanished, it did so only to reappear in terms of another. But one step more was necessary to complete this magnificent theory. What can produce motion but motion itself? Into what can motion be converted, but motion? May not these forces, thus mutually convertible, be simply different modes of motion of the molecules of matter, precisely as mechanical motion is a motion of its mass? Thus was born the dynamic theory of force, first brought out in any completeness by Mr. Grove, in 1842, in a lecture on the "Progress of Physical Science," delivered at the London Institution. In that lecture he said: "Light, heat, electricity, magnetism, motion, are all convertible material affections. Assuming either as the cause, one of the others will be the effect. Thus heat may be said to produce electricity, electricity to produce heat; magnetism to produce electricity, electricity magnetism; and so of the rest."[8]

A few simple experiments will help us to fix in our minds the great fact of the convertibility of force. Starting with actual visible motion, correlation requires that when it disappears as motion, it should reappear as heat, light, or electricity. If the moving body be elastic like this rubber ball, then its motion is not destroyed when it strikes, but is only changed in direction. But if it be non-elastic, like this ball of lead, then it does not rebound; its motion is converted into heat. The motion of this sledge-hammer, for example, which if received upon this anvil would be simply changed in direction, if allowed to fall upon this bar of lead, is converted into heat; the evidence of which is that a piece of phosphorus placed upon the lead is at once inflamed. So too, if motion be arrested by the cushion of air in this cylinder, the heat evolved fires the tinder carried in the plunger. But it is not necessary that the arrest of motion should be sudden; it may be gradual, as in the case of friction. If this cylinder containing water or alcohol be caused to revolve rapidly between the two sides of this wooden rubber, the heat due to the arrested motion will raise the temperature of the liquid to the boiling point, and the cork will be expelled. But motion may also be converted into electricity. Indeed electricity is always the result of friction between heterogeneous particles.[9] When this piece of hard rubber, for example, is rubbed with the fur of a cat, it is at once electrified ; and now if it be caused to communicate a portion of its charge to this glass plate, to which at the same time we add the mechanical motion of rotation, the strong sparks produced give evidence of the conversion.

So, too, taking heat as the initial force, motion, light, electricity may be produced. In every steam-engine the steam which leaves the cylinder is cooler than that which entered it, and cooler by exactly the amount of work done. The motion of the piston's mass is precisely that lost by the steam molecules which batter against it. The conversion of heat into electricity, too, is also easily effected. When the junction of two metals is heated, electricity is developed. If the two metals be bismuth and antimony, as represented in this diagram, the currents flow as indicated by the arrows ; and by multiplying the number of pairs, the effect may be proportionately increased. Such an arrangement, called a thermo-electric battery, we have here ; and by it the heat of a single gas-burner may be made to move, when converted, this little electric bell-engine. Moreover, heat and light have the very closest analogy ; exalt the rapidity with which the molecules move and light appears, the difference being only one of intensity.

Again, if electricity be our starting point, we may accomplish its conversion into the other forces. Heat results whenever its passage is interrupted or resisted; a wire of the poorly conducting metal platinum becoming even red hot by the converted electricity. To produce light, of course, we need only to intensify this action; the brightest artificial light known, results from a direct conversion of electricity.

Enough has now been said to establish our point. What is to be particularly observed of these pieces of apparatus is that they are machines especially designed for the conversion of some one force into another. And we expect of them only that conversion. We pass on to consider for a moment the quantitative relations of this mutual convertibility. We notice, in the first place, that in all cases save one, the conversion is not perfect, a part of the force used not being utilized, on the one hand, and on the other, other forces making their appearance simultaneously. While, for example, the conversion of motion into heat is quite complete, the inverse conversion is not at all so. And on the other hand, when motion is converted into electricity, a part of it appears as heat. This simultaneous production of many forces is well illustrated by our little bell-engine, which converts the electricity of the thermo-battery into magnetism, and this into motion, a part of which expends itself as sound. For these reasons the question "How much?" is one not easily answered in all cases. The best known of these relations is that between motion and heat, which was first established by Mr. Joule in 1849, after seven years of patient investigation.[10] The apparatus which he used is shown in the diagram. It consists of a cylindrical box of metal, through the cover of which passes a shaft, carrying upon its lower end a set of paddles, immersed in water within the box, and upon its upper portion a drum, on which are wound two cords, which, passing in opposite directions, run over pulleys, and are attached to known weights. The temperature of the water within the box being carefully noted, the weights are then allowed to fall a certain number of times, of course in their fall turning the paddles against the friction of the liquid. At the close of the experiment the water is found to be warmer than before. And by measuring the amount of this rise in temperature, knowing the distance through which the weights have fallen, it is easy to calculate the quantity of heat which corresponds to a given amount of motion. In this way, and as a mean of a large number of experiments, Mr. Joule found that the amount of mass motion in a body weighing one pound, which had fallen from a hight of 772 feet, was exactly equal to the molecular motion which must be added to a pound of water, in order to heat it one degree Fahrenheit. If we call the actual energy of a body weighing one pound which has fallen one foot, a foot-pound, then we may speak of the mechanical equivalent of heat as being 772 foot-pounds.

The significance and value of this numerical constant will appear more clearly if we apply it to the solution of one or two simple problems. During the recent war two immense iron guns were cast in Pittsburgh, whose weight was nearly 112,000 pounds each, and which had a caliber of 20 inches.[11] Upon this diagram is a calculation of the effective blow which the solid shot of such a gun, assuming its weight to be 1,000 pounds and its velocity 1,100 feet per second, would give; it is 902,797 tons![12] Now, if it were possible to convert the whole of this enormous mechanical power into heat, to how much would it correspond? This question may be answered by the aid of the mechanical equivalent of heat; here is the calculation, from which we see that when 17 gallons of ice-cold water are heated to the boiling point, as much energy is communicated as is contained in the death-dealing missile at its highest velocity.[13] Again, if we take the impact of a larger cannon-ball, our earth, which is whirling through space with a velocity of 19 miles a second, we find it to be 98,416,136,000,000,000,000,000,000,000,000 tons![14] Were this energy all converted into heat, it would equal that produced by the combustion of 14 earths of solid coal.[15]

The conversion of heat into motion, however, as already stated, is not as perfect. The best steam-engines economize only one-twentieth of the heat of the fuel.[16] Hence if a steamship require 600 tons of coal to carry her across the Atlantic, 570 tons will be expended in heating the waters of the ocean, the heat of the remaining 30 tons only being converted into work.

One other quantitative determination of force has also been made. Prof. Julius Thomsen, of Copenhagen, has fixed experimentally the mechanical equivalent of light.[17] He finds that the energy of the light of a spermaceti candle burning 126½ grains per hour, is equal in mechanical value to 13·1 foot-pounds per minute. The same conclusion has been reached by Mr. Farmer, of Boston, from different data.[18]

If we pass from the actual physical energies or motions to consider for a moment the potential energies or attractions, we find, also, an intimate correlation. Since all energy not active in motion is potential in attraction, it follows that in the attractions we have energy stored up for subsequent use. The sun is thus storing up energy: every minute it raises 2,000,000,000 tons of water to the mean hight of the clouds, 3½ miles; and the actual energy set free when this water falls is equal to 2,757,000,000,000 horse powers.[19] So when the oxygen and the zinc of the ore are separated in the furnace, the actual energy of heat becomes the potential energy of chemical attraction, which again becomes actual in the form of electricity when the zinc is dissolved in an acid. We see, then, that not only may any form of force or actual energy be stored up as any form of attraction or potential energy, but that the latter, from whatsoever source derived, may appear as heat, light, electricity, or mechanical motion.

Having now established the fact of correlation for the physical forces, we have next to inquire what are the evidences of the correlation of the vital forces with them. But in the first place it must be remarked that life is not a simple term like heat or electricity; it is a complex term, and includes all those phenomena which a living body exhibits. In this discussion, therefore, we shall use the term vital force to express only the actual energy of the body, however manifested. As to the attractions or the potential energy of the organism, nothing is more fully settled in science than the fact that these are precisely the same within the body as without it. Every particle of matter within the body obeys implicitly the laws of the chemical and physical attractions. No overpowering or supernatural agency comes in to complicate their action, which is modified only by the action of the others. Vitality, therefore, is the sum of the energies of a living body, both potential and actual.

Moreover, the important fact must be fully recognized that in living beings we have to do with no new elementary forms of matter. Precisely the same atoms which build up the inorganic fabric, compose the organic. In the early days of chemistry, indeed, it was supposed that the complicated molecules which life produced were beyond the reach of simple chemical law. But as more and more complex molecules have been, one after another, produced, chemistry has become re-assured, and now doubts not her ability to produce them all. A few years hence, and she will doubtless give us quinine and protagon, as she now gives us coumarin and neurine, substances the synthesis of which was but yesterday an impossibility.[20]

In studying the phenomena of living beings, it is important also to bear in mind the different and at the same time the coördinate purposes subserved by the two great kingdoms of nature. The food of the plant is matter whose energy is all expended; it is a fallen weight. But the plant-organism receives it, exposes it to the sun's ray, and, in a way yet mysterious to us, converts the actual energy of the sunlight into potential energy within it. The fallen weight is thus raised, and energy is stored up in substances which now are alone competent to become the food of the animal. This food is not such because any new atoms have been added to it; it is food because it contains within it potential energy, which at any time may become actual as force. This food the animal now appropriates ; he brings it in contact with oxygen, and the potential energy becomes actual ; he cuts the string, the weight falls, and what was just now only attraction, has become actual force ; this force he uses for his own purposes, and hands back the oxidized matter, the fallen weight, to the plant to be again de-oxidized, to be again raised. The plant then is to regarded as a machine for converting sunlight into potential energy ; the animal, a machine for setting the potential energy free as actual, and economizing it. The force which the plant stores up is undeniably physical ; must not the force which the animal sets free by its conversion, be intimately correlated to it?

But approaching our question still more closely, let us, in illustration of the vital forces of the animal economy, choose three forms of its manifestation in which to seek for the evidences of correlation ; these shall be heat, evolved within the body ; muscular energy or motion ; and lastly, nervous energy, or that form of force which, on the one hand, stimulates a muscle to contract, and on the other, appears in forms called mental.

The heat which is produced by the living body is obviously of the same nature as heat from any other source ; it is recognized by the same tests, and may be applied for the same purposes. As to its origin, it is evident that since potential energy exists in the food which enters the body, and is there converted into force, a portion of it may become the actual energy of heat. And since, too, the heat produced in the body is precisely such as would be set free by the combustion of this food outside of it, it is fair to assume that it thus originates. To this may be added the chemical argument that while food capable of yielding heat by combustion is taken into the body, its constituents are completely or almost completely, oxidized before leaving it; and since oxidation always evolves heat, the heat of the body must have its origin in the oxidation of the food. Moreover, careful measurements have demonstrated that the amount of heat given off by the body of a man weighing 180 pounds is about 2,500,000 units. Accurate calculations have shown, on the other hand, that 288·4 grams of carbon and 12·56 grams of hydrogen are available in the daily food for the production of heat. If burned out of the body, these quantities of carbon and hydrogen would yield 2,765,134 heat units. Burned within it, as we have just seen, 2,500,000 units appear as heat; the rest in other forms of energy.[21] We conceive, however, that no long argument is necessary to prove that animal heat results from a conversion of energy within the body; or that the vital force heat, is as truly correlated to the other forces as when it it has a purely physical origin.

The belief that the muscular force exerted by an animal is created by him is by no means confined to the very earliest ages of history. Traces of it appear to the careful observer even now, although, as Dr. Frankland says, science has proved that "an animal can no more generate an amount of force capable of moving a grain of sand than a stone can fall upward or a locomotive drive a train without fuel."[22] In studying the characters of muscular action we notice, first, that, as in the case of heat, the force which it develops is in no wise different from motion in inorganic nature. In the early part of the lecture, motion produced by the contraction of muscle, was used to show the conversion of mass-force into molecular force. No one in this room believes, I presume, that the result would have been at all different, had the motion been supplied by a steam-engine or a water-wheel. Again, food, as we have seen, is of value for the potential energy it contains, which may become actual in the body. Liebig, in 1842, asserted that for the production of muscular force, the food must first be converted into muscular tissue,[23] a view until recently accepted by physiologists.[24] It has been conclusively shown, however, within a few years, that muscular force cannot come from the oxidation of its own substance, since the products of this metamorphosis are not increased in amount by muscular exertion.[25] Indeed, reasoning from the whole amount of such products excreted, the oxidation of the amount of muscle which they represent would furnish scarcely one-fifth of the mechanical force of the body. But while the products of tissue-oxidation do not increase with the increase of muscular exertion, the amount of carbonic gas exhaled by the lungs is increased in the exact ratio of the work done.[26] No doubt can be entertained, therefore, that the actual energy of the muscle is simply the converted potential energy of the carbon of the food. A muscle, therefore, like a steam-engine, is a machine for converting the potential energy of carbon into motion. But unlike a steam-engine, the muscle accomplishes this conversion directly, the energy not passing through the intermediate stage of heat. For this reason, the muscle is the most economical producer of mechanical force known. While no machine whatever can transform all of the energy into motion—the most economical steam engines utilizing only one-twentieth of the heat—the muscle is able to convert one-fifth of the energy of the food into work.[27] The other four-fifths must, therefore, appear as heat. Whenever a muscle contracts, then, four times as much energy appears as heat as is converted into motion. Direct experiments by Heidenhain have confirmed this, by showing that an important rise of temperature attends muscular contraction;[28] a fact, however, apparent to any one who has ever taken active exercise. The work done by the animal body is of two sorts, internal and external. The former includes the action of the heart, of the respiratory muscles, and of those assisting the digestive process. The latter refers to the useful work the body may perform. Careful estimates place the entire work of the body at about 800 foot-tons daily; of which 450 foot-tons is internal, 350 foot-tons external work. And since the internal work ultimately appears as heat within the body, the actual loss of heat by the production of motion is the equivalent of the 350 foot-tons which represents external work. This by a simple calculation will be found to be 250,000 heat units, almost the precise amount by which the heat yielded by the food when burned without the body, exceeds that actually evolved by the organism. Moreover, while the total heat given off by the body is 2,500,000 units, the amount of energy evolved as work is equal to about 600,000 heat units; hence the amount of work done by a muscle is as above stated, one-fifth of the actual energy derivable from the food. One point further. The law of correlation requires that the heat set free when a muscle in contracting does work, shall be less than when it effects nothing; this fact, too, has been experimentally established by Heidenhain.[29] So, again, when muscular contraction does not result in motion, as when one tries to raise a weight too heavy for him, the energy which would have appeared as work, takes the form of heat: a result deducible by the law of correlation from the steam-engine.

The last of the so-called vital forces which we are to examine, is that produced by the nerves and nervous centers. In the nerve which stimulates a muscle to contract, this force is undeniably motion, since it is propagated along this nerve from one extremity to the other. In common language, too, this idea finds currency in the comparison of this force to electricity; the gray or cellular matter being the battery, the white or fibrous matter the conductors. That this force is not electricity, however, Du Bois-Reymond has demonstrated by showing that its velocity is only 97 feet in a second, a speed equaled by the greyhound and the race-horse.[30] In his opinion, the propagation of a nervous impulse is a sort of successive molecular polarization, like magnetism. But that this agent is a force, as analogous to electricity as is magnetism, is shown not only by the fact that the transmission of electricity along a nerve will cause the contraction of the muscle to which it leads, but also by the more important fact that the contraction of a muscle is excited by diminishing its normal electrical current;[31] a result which could take place only with a stimulus closely allied to electricity. Nerve-force, therefore, must be a transmuted potential energy.

What, now, shall we say of that highest manifestation of animal life, thought-power? Has the upper region called intelligence and reason, any relations to physical force? This realm has not escaped the searching investigation of modern science; and although in it investigations are vastly more difficult than in any of the regions thus far considered, yet some results of great value have been obtained, which may help us to a solution of our problem. It is to be observed at the outset that every external manifestation of thought-force is a muscular one, as a word spoken or written, a gesture, or an expression of the face; and hence this force must be intimately correlated with nerve-force. These manifestations, reaching the mind through the avenues of sense, awaken accordant trains of thought only when this muscular evidence is understood. A blank sheet of paper excites no emotion; even covered with Assyrian cuneiform characters, its alternations of black and white awaken no response in the ordinary brain. It is only when, by a frequent repetition of these impressions, the brain-cell has been educated, that these before meaningless characters awaken thought. Is thought, then, simply a cell action which may or may not result in muscular expression—an action which originates new combinations of truth only, precisely as a calculating machine evolves new combinations of figures? Whatever we define thought to be, this fact appears certain, that it is capable of external manifestation by conversion into the actual energy of motion, and only by this conversion. But here the question arises, Can it be manifested inwardly without such a transformation of energy? Or is the evolution of thought entirely independent of the matter of the brain? Experiments, ingenious and reliable, have answered this question. The importance of the results will, I trust, warrant me in examining the methods employed in these experiments somewhat in detail. Inasmuch as our methods for measuring minute amounts of electricity are very perfect, and the methods for the conversion of heat into electricity are equally delicate, it has been found that smaller differences of temperature may be recognized by converting the heat into electricity, than can be detected thermometrically. The apparatus, first used by Melloni in 1832,[32] is very simple, consisting first, of a pair of metallic bars like those described in the early part of the lecture, for effecting the conversion of the heat; and second, of a delicate galvanometer, for measuring the electricity produced. In the experiments in question one of the bars used was made of bismuth, the other of an alloy of antimony and zinc.[33] Preliminary trials having shown that any change of temperature within the skull was soonest manifested externally in that depression which exists just above the occipital protuberance, a pair of these little bars was fastened to the head at this point; and to neutralize the results of a general rise of temperature over the whole body, a second pair, reversed in direction, was attached to the leg or arm, so that if a like increase of heat came to both, the electricity developed by one would be neutralized by the other, and no effect be produced upon the needle unless only one was affected. By long practice it was ascertained that a state of mental torpor could be induced, lasting for hours, in which the needle remained stationary. But let a person knock on the door outside the room, or speak a single word, even though the experimenter remained absolutely passive, and the reception of the intelligence caused the needle to swing through 20 degrees.[34] In explanation of this production of heat, the analogy of the muscle at once suggests itself. No conversion of energy is complete; and as the heat of muscular action represents force which has escaped conversion into motion, so the heat evolved during the reception of an idea, is energy which has escaped conversion into thought, from precisely the same cause. Moreover, these experiments have shown that ideas which affect the emotions, produce most heat in their reception; "a few minutes' recitation to one's self of emotional poetry, producing more effect than several hours of deep thought." Hence it is evident that the mechanism for the production of deep thought, accomplishes this conversion of energy far more perfectly than that which produces simply emotion. But we may take a step further in this same direction. A muscle, precisely as the law of correlation requires, develops less heat when doing work than when it contracts without doing it. Suppose, now, that beside the simple reception of an idea by the brain, the thought is expressed outwardly by some muscular sign. The conversion now takes two directions, and in addition to the production of thought, a portion of the energy appears as nerve and muscle-power; less, therefore, should appear as heat, according to our law of correlation. Dr. Lombard's experiments have shown that the amount of heat developed by the recitation to one's self of emotional poetry, was in every case less when that recitation was oral; *i. e.*, had a muscular expression. These results are in accordance with the well-known fact that emotion often finds relief in physical demonstrations; thus diminishing the emotional energy by converting it into muscular.

Nor do these facts rest upon physical evidence alone. Chemistry teaches that thought-force, like muscle-force, comes from the food ; and demonstrates that the force evolved by the brain, like that produced by the muscle, comes not from the disintegration of its own tissue, but is the converted energy of burning carbon.[35] Can we longer doubt, then, that the brain, too, is a machine for the conversion of energy? Can we longer refuse to believe that even thought is, in some mysterious way, correlated to the other natural forces? and this, even in face of the fact that it has never yet been measured?[36]

I cannot close without saying a word concerning the part which our own country has had in the development of these great truths. Beginning with heat, we find that the material theory of caloric is indebted for its overthrow more to the distinguished Count Rumford than to any other one man. While superintending the boring of cannon at the Munich Arsenal towards the close of the last century, he was struck by the large amount of heat developed, and instituted a careful series of experiments to ascertain its origin. These experiments led him to the conclusion that "anything which any insulated body or system of bodies can continue to furnish without limitation, cannot possibly be a material substance." But this man, to whom must be ascribed the discovery of the first great law of the correlation of energy, was an American. Born in Woburn, Mass., in 1753, he, under the name of Benjamin Thompson, taught school afterward at Concord, N. H., then called Rumford. Unjustly suspected of toryism during our Revolutionary war, he went abroad and distinguished himself in the service of several of the Governments of

Europe. He did not forget his native land, though she had treated him so unfairly; when the honor of knighthood was tendered him, he chose as his title the name of the Yankee village where he had taught school, and was thenceforward known as Count Rumford. And at his death, by founding a professorship in Harvard College, and donating a prize-fund to the American Academy of Arts and Sciences at Boston, he showed his interest in her prosperity and advancement.[37] Nor has the field of vital forces been without earnest workers belonging to our own country. Professors John W. Draper[38] and Joseph Henry[39] were among its earliest explorers. And in 1851, Dr. J. H. Watters, now of St. Louis, published a theory of the origin of vital force, almost identical with that for which Dr. Carpenter, of London, has of late received so much credit. Indeed, there is some reason to believe that Dr. Watters's essay may have suggested to the distinguished English physiologist the germs of his own theory.[40] A paper on this subject by Prof. Joseph Leconte, of Columbia, S. C., published in 1859, attracted much attention abroad.[41] The remarkable results already given on the relation of heat to mental work, which thus far are unique in science, we owe to Professor J. S. Lombard, of Harvard College;[42] the very combination of metals used in his apparatus being devised by our distinguished electrical engineer, Mr. Moses G. Farmer. Finally, researches conducted by Dr. T. R. Noyes in the Physiological Laboratory of Yale College, have confirmed the theory that muscular tissue does not wear during action, up to the point of fatigue;[43] and other researches by Dr. L. H. Wood have first established the same great truth for brain-tissue.[44]

We need not be ashamed, then, of our part in this advance in science. Our workers are, indeed, but few; but both they and their results will live in the records of the world's progress. More would there be now of them were such studies more fostered and encouraged. Self-denying, earnest men are ready to give themselves up to the solution of these problems, if only the means of a bare subsistence be allowed them. When wealth shall foster science, science will increase wealth—wealth pecuniary, it is true: but also wealth of knowledge, which is far better.

In looking back over the whole of this discussion, I trust that it is possible to see that the objects which we had in view at its commencement have been more or less fully attained. I would fain believe that we now see more clearly the beautiful harmonies of bounteous nature; that on her many-stringed instrument force answers to force, like the notes of a great symphony; disappearing now in potential energy, and anon reappearing as actual energy, in a multitude of forms. I would hope that this wonderful unity and mutual interaction of force in the dead forms of inorganic nature, appears to you identical in the living forms of animal and vegetable life, which make of our earth an Eden. That even that mysterious, and in many aspects awful, power of thought, by which man influences the present and future ages, is a part of this great ocean of energy. But here the great question rolls upon us, Is it only this? Is there not behind this material substance, a higher than molecular power in the thoughts which are immortalized in the poetry of a Milton or a Shakespeare, the art creations of a Michael Angelo or a Titian, the harmonies of a Mozart or a Beethoven? Is there really no immortal portion separable from this brain-tissue, though yet mysteriously united to it? In a word, does this curiously-fashioned body inclose a soul, God-given and to God returning? Here Science veils her face and bows in reverence before the Almighty. We have passed the boundaries by which physical science is inclosed. No crucible, no subtle magnetic needle can answer now our questions. No word but His who formed us, can break the awful silence. In presence of such a revelation Science is dumb, and faith comes in joyfully to accept that higher truth which can never be the object of physical demonstration.

NOTES AND REFERENCES.

---

1 HUMBOLDT, Views of Nature, Bohn's ed., London, 1850, p. 380. This allegory did not appear in the first edition of the Views of Nature. In the preface to the second edition the author gives the following account of its origin: "Schiller," he says, "in remembrance of his youthful medical studies, loved to converse with me, during my long stay at Jena, on physiological subjects." * * * "It was at this period that I wrote the little allegory on Vital Force, called The Rhodian Genius. The predilection which Schiller entertained for this piece, which he admitted into his periodical, *Die Horen*, gave me courage to introduce it here." It was published in *Die Horen* in 1795.

2 HUMBOLDT, *op. cit.*, p. 386. In his *Aphorismi ex doctrina Physiologiæ chemicæ Plantarum*, appended to his *Flora Fribergensis subterranea*, published in 1793, Humboldt had said "Vim internam, quæ chymicæ affinitatis vincula resolvit, atque obstat, quominus elementa corporum libere conjungantur, vitalem vocamus." "That internal force, which dissolves the bonds of chemical affinity, and prevents the elements of bodies from freely uniting, we call vital." But in a note to the allegory above mentioned, added to the third edition of the Views of Nature in 1849, he says: "Reflection and prolonged study in the departments of physiology and chemistry have deeply shaken my earlier belief in peculiar so-called vital forces. In the year 1797, * * * I already declared that I by no means regarded the existence of these peculiar vital forces as established." And again: "The difficulty of satisfactorily referring the vital phe-

nomena of the organism to physical and chemical laws depends chiefly (and almost in the same manner as the prediction of meteorological processes in the atmosphere) on the complication of the phenomena, and on the great number of the simultaneously acting forces as well as the conditions of their activity."

3 Compare HENRY BENCE JONES, Croonian Lectures on Matter and Force. London, 1868, John Churchill & Sons.

4 Ib., Preface, p. vi.

5 RANKINE, W. J. M., Philosophical Magazine, Feb., 1853. Also Edinburgh Philosophical Journal, July, 1855.

6 ARMSTRONG, Sir WM. In his address as President of the British Association for the Advancement of Science. Rep. Brit. Assoc., 1863, li.

7 GROVE, W. R., in 1842. Compare "Nature" i, 335, Jan. 27, 1870. Also Appleton's Journal, iii, 324, Mch. 19, 1870.

8 Id., in Preface to The Correlation of Physical Forces, 4th ed. Reprinted in The Correlation and Conservation of Forces, edited by E. L. Youmans, p. 7. New York, 1865, D. Appleton & Co.

9 Id., ib., Am. ed., p. 33 et seq.

10 JOULE, J. P., Philosophical Transactions, 1850, p. 61.

11 See American Journal of Science, II, xxxvii, 296, 1864.

12 The work (W) done by a moving body is commonly expressed by the formula $W=MV^2$, in which M, or the mass of the body, is equal to $\frac{w}{2g}$; *i. e.*, to the weight divided by twice the intensity of gravity. The work done by our cannon-ball then, would be $\frac{1\times(1100)^2}{2\times64\frac{1}{3}}$=9,404·14 foot-tons. If, further, we assume the resisting body to be of such a character as to bring the ball to rest in moving $\frac{1}{4}$ of an inch, then the final pressure would be 9,404·14×12×4=451,398·7 tons. But since, "in the case of a prefectly elastic body, or of a resistance proportional to the advance of the center of gravity of the impinging body from the point at which contact first takes place, the final pressure (provided the body

struck is perfectly rigid) is double what would occur were the stoppage to occur at the end of a corresponding advance against a uniform resistance," this result must be multiplied by two; and we get (451,398·7×2) 902,797 tons as the crushing pressure of the ball under these conditions. [The author's thanks are due to his friends Pres. F. A. P. Barnard and Mr. J. J. Skinner for suggestions on the relation of impact to statical pressure.]

13 The unit of impact being that given by a body weighing one pound and moving one foot a second, the impact of such a body falling from a hight of 772 feet—the velocity acquired being 222¼ feet per second ($=\sqrt{2sg}$)—would be $1\times(222\frac{1}{4})^2=49,408$ units, the equivalent in impact of one heat-unit. A cannon-ball weighing 1000 lbs. and moving 1100 feet a second would have an impact of $(1100)^2\times1000=1,210,000,000$ units. Dividing this by 49,408, the quotient is 24489 heat-units, the equivalent of the impact. The specific heat of iron being ·1138, this amount of heat would raise the temperature of one pound of iron 215,191° F. (24,489×·1138) or of 1000 pounds of iron 215° F. 24489 pounds of water heated one degree, is equal to 136½ pounds, or 17 gallons U. S., heated 180 degrees; *i. e.*, from 32° to 212° F.

14 Assuming the density of the earth to be 5·5, its weight would be 6,500,000,000,000,000,000,000 tons, and its impact—by the formula given above—would be 1,025,000,000,000,000,000,000,000,000,000 foot-tons. Making the same supposition as in the case of our cannon-ball, the final pressure would be that here stated.

15 TYNDALL, J., Heat considered as a mode of Motion, Am. ed., p. 57, New York, 1863.

16 RANKINE (The Steam-engine and other prime Movers, London, 1866,) gives the efficiency of Steam-engines as from 1-15th to 1-20th of the heat of the fuel.

ARMSTRONG, Sir WM., places this efficiency at 1-10th as the maximum. In practice, the average result is only 1-30th. Rep. Brit. Assoc., 1863, p. liv.

HELMHOLTZ, H. L. F., says: "The best expansive engines give back as mechanical work only eighteen per cent. of the heat generated by the fuel." Interaction of Natural Forces, in Correlation and Conservation of Forces, p. 227.

17 THOMSEN, JULIUS, Poggendorff's Annalen, cxxv, 348. Also in abstract in Am. J. Sci., II, xli, 396, May, 1866.

18 American Journal of Science, II, xli, 214, March, 1866.

19 In this calculation the annual evaporation from the ocean is assumed to be about 9 feet. (See Dr. BUIST, quoted in Maury's Phys. Geography of the Sea, New York, 1861, p. 11.) Calling the water-area of our globe 150,000,000 square miles, the total evaporation in tons per minute, would be that here given. Inasmuch as 30,000 pounds raised one-foot high is a horse-power, the number of horse-powers necessary to raise this quantity of water 3½ miles in one minute is 2,757,000,000,000. This amount of energy is precisely that set free again when this water falls as rain.

20 Compare ODLING, WM., Lectures on Animal Chemistry, London, 1866. "In broad antagonism to the doctrines which only a few years back were regarded as indisputable, we now find that the chemist, like the plant, is capable of producing from carbonic acid and water a whole host of organic bodies, and we see no reason to question his ultimate ability to reproduce all animal and vegetable principles whatsoever." (p. 52.)

"Already hundreds of organic principles have been built up from their constituent elements, and there is now no reason to doubt our capability of producing all organic principles whatsoever in a similar manner." (p. 58.)

Dr. Odling is the successor of Faraday as Fullerian Professor of Chemistry in the Royal Institution of Great Britain.

21 MARSHALL, JOHN, Outlines of Physiology, American edition, 1868, p. 916.

22 FRANKLAND, EDWARD, On the Source of Muscular Power, Proc. Roy. Inst., June 8, 1866; Am. J. Sci., II, xlii, 393, Nov. 1866.

23 LIEBIG, JUSTUS VON, Die organische Chemie in ihrer Anwendung auf Physiologie und Pathologie, Braunschweig, 1842. Also in his Animal Chemistry, edition of 1852 (Am. ed., p. 26), where he says "Every motion increases the amount of organized tissue which undergoes metamorphosis."

24 Compare DRAPER, JOHN WM. Human Physiology.

PLAYFAIR, LYON, On the Food of Man in relation to his useful work, Edinburgh, 1865. Proc. Roy. Inst., Apr. 28, 1865.

RANKE, Tetanus eine Physiologische Studie, Leipzig, 1865.

ODLING, *op. cit.*

25 VOIT, E., Untersuchungen über den Einfluss des Kochsalzes, des Kaffees, und der Muskelbewegungen auf den Stoffwechsel, Munich, 1860.

SMITH, E., Philosophical Transactions, 1861, 747.

FICK, A., and WISLICENUS, J., Phil. Mag., IV, xxxi, 485.

FRANKLAND, E., *loc. cit.*

NOYES, T. R., American Journal Medical Sciences, Oct. 1867.

PARKES, E. A., Proceedings Royal Society, xv, 339; xvi, 44.

26 SMITH, EDWARD, Philosophical Transactions, 1859, 709.

27 Authorities differ as to the amount of energy converted by the steam-engine. (See Note 16.) Compare MARSHALL, *op. cit.*, p. 918. "Whilst, therefore, in an engine one-twentieth part only of the fuel consumed is utilized as mechanical power, one-fifth of the food absorbed by man is so appropriated."

28 HEIDENHAIN, Mechanische Leistung Wärmeentwickelung und Stoffumsatz bei der Muskelthätigkeit, Breslau, 1864.

See also HAUGHTON, SAMUEL, On the Relation of Food to work, published in "Medicine in Modern Times," London, 1869, Macmillan & Co.

29 HEIDENHAIN, *op. cit.* Also by FICK, Untersuchungen über Muskel-arbeit, Basel, 1867. Compare also "Nature," i, 159, Dec. 9, 1869.

30 DU BOIS-REYMOND, EMIL, On the time required for the transmission of volition and sensation through the nerves, Proc. Roy. Inst. Also in Appendix to Bence Jones's Croonian lectures.

31 MARSHALL, *op. cit.*, p. 227.

32 MELLONI, Ann. Ch. Phys., xlviii, 198.

See also NOBILI, Bibl. Univ., xliv, 225, 1830; lvii, 1, 1834.

33 The apparatus employed is illustrated and fully described in Brown-Sequard's Archives de Physiologie, i, 498, June, 1868. By it the 1-4000th of a degree Centigrade may be indicated.

34 LOMBARD, J. S., New York Medical Journal, v, 198, June, 1867. [A part of these facts were communicated to me directly by their discoverer.]

35 WOOD, L. H., On the influence of Mental activity on the Excretion of Phosphoric acid by the Kidneys. Proceedings Connecticut Medical Society for 1869, p. 197.

36 On this question of vital force, see LIEBIG, Animal Chemistry. "The increase of mass in a plant is determined by the occurrence of a decomposition which takes place in certain parts of the plant under the influence of light and heat."

"The modern science of Physiology has left the track of Aristotle. To the eternal advantage of science, and to the benefit of mankind it no longer invents a *horror vacui*, a *quinta essentia*, in order to furnish credulous hearers with solutions and explanations of phenomena, whose true connection with others, whose ultimate cause is still unknown."

"All the parts of the animal body are produced from a peculiar fluid circulating in its organism, by virtue of an influence residing in every cell, in every organ, or part of an organ."

"Physiology has sufficiently decisive grounds for the opinion that every motion, every manifestation of force, is the result of a transformation of the structure or of its substance; that every conception, every mental affection, is followed by changes in the chemical nature of the secreted fluids; that every thought, every sensation is accompanied by a change in the composition of the substance of the brain."

"All vital activity arises from the mutual action of the oxygen of the atmosphere and the elements of the food."

"As, in the closed galvanic circuit, in consequence of certain changes which an inorganic body, a metal, undergoes when placed in contact with an acid, a certain something becomes cognizable by our senses, which we call a current of electricity; so in the animal body, in consequence of transformations and changes undergone by matter previously constituting a part of the organism, certain phenomena of motion and activity are perceived, and these we call life, or vitality."

"In the animal body we recognize as the ultimate cause of all force only one cause, the chemical action which the elements of the food and the oxygen of the air mutually exercise on each other. The only known ultimate cause of vital force, either in animals or in plants, is a chemical process."

"If we consider the force which determines the vital phenomena as a property of certain substances, this view leads of itself to a new and more rigorous consideration of certain singular phenomena, which these very substances exhibit, in circumstances in which they no longer make a part of living organisms."

Also OWEN, RICHARD, (Derivative Hypothesis of Life and Species, forming the 40th chapter of his Anatomy of Vertebrates, republished in Am. J. Sci., II, xlvii, 33, Jan. 1869.) "In the endeavor to clearly comprehend and explain the functions of the combination of forces called 'brain,' the physiologist is hindered and troubled by the views of the nature of those cerebral forces which the needs of dogmatic theology have imposed on mankind." * * "Religion pure and undefiled, can best answer how far it is righteous or just to charge a neighbor with being unsound in his principles who holds the term 'life' to be a sound expressing the sum of living phenomena; and who maintains these phenomena to be modes of force into which other forms of force have passed, from potential to active states, and reciprocally, through the agency of these sums or combinations of forces impressing the mind with the ideas signified by the terms 'monad,' 'moss,' 'plant,' or 'animal.'"

And HUXLEY, THOS. H., "On the Physical Basis of Life," University Series, No. 1. College Courant, 1870.

Per contra, see the Address of Dr. F. A. P. Barnard, as retiring President, before the Am. Assoc. for the Advancement of Science, Chicago meeting, August, 1868. "Thought cannot be a physical force, because thought admits of no measure."

GOULD, BENJ. APTHORP, Address as retiring President, before the American Association at its Salem meeting, Aug., 1869.

BEALE, LIONEL S., "Protoplasm, or Life, Matter, and Mind." London, 1870. John Churchill & Sons.

37 For an excellent account of this distinguished man, see Youmans's Introduction to the Correlation and Conservation of Forces, p. xvii.

38 DRAPER, J. W., *loc. cit.*

39 HENRY, JOSEPH, Agric. Rep. Patent Office, 1857, 440.

40 WATTERS, J. H., An Essay on Organic, or Life-force. Written for the degree of Doctor of Medicine in the University of Pennsylvania, Philadelphia, 1851. See also St. Louis Medical and Surgical Journal, II, v, Nos. 3 and 4, 1868; Dec. 1868, and Nov. 10, 1869.

41 LECONTE, JOSEPH, The Correlation of Physical, Chemical and Vital Force, and the Conservation of Force in Vital Phenomena. American Journal of Science, II, xxviii, 305, Nov. 1859.

42 LOMBARD, J. S., *loc. cit.*

43 NOYES, T. R., *loc. cit.*

44 WOOD, L. H., *loc. cit.*

www.ingramcontent.com/pod-product-compliance
Lightning Source LLC
LaVergne TN
LVHW012329100826
845148LV00017B/674